HEART DISEASE
A NEW DIRECTION

Dr. Ramesh I. Kapadia

Foreword
Dr. B. M. Hegde,
M.D., F.R.C.P. (London); F.R.C.P. (Edin.),

F.R.C.P. (Glasgo); F.A.C.C.

Navajivan Publishing House
Ahmedabad-380 014

Rupees 25/-

© Dr. Ramesh I. Kapadia, 2001
36, Jain Society, Ellisbridge,
Ahmedabad-380 006
India

Email : rikapadia@icenet.net
www : universalhealing.org

First Edition : 2,000 Copies, October 1995
Second Reprint : 1,000 Copies, April 2003
Total : 5,000 Copies

ISBN 81-7229-132-9

Printed and Published by
Jitendra T. Desai
Navajivan Publishing House
Ahmedabad-380 014
India

For
The Participants of
Universal Healing Program

FOREWORD

Reductionist science of specialities has been responsible for the sorry state of affairs in modern medicine today. Modern medicine, with all the tools, has not only become inhuman but seems to have lost its sense of direction. Science is heading for a crisis, while the new science of *CHAOS* is trying to save mankind. Human body is a dynamic machine run by the mind and is constantly being fuelled by food and oxygen. The linear Euclidean mathematical rules of conventional sciences do not apply to the human organism. The conventional risk factor hypotheses have been proven wrong time and again. The pooling Project Data have shown that while only 10% of those with more than six risk factors eventually had a heart attack, 60% of those who had a heart attack did have ONE or NONE of the conventional risk factors operating in them. Still we hang on to the old theories.

Mind runs the body, and the connection between the two is so intimate, that it is difficult to separate one from the other. Anger is now shown to be the greatest risk factor for stroke and even heart attacks. Heart rate variability is common in children; as age advances it gradually becomes less obvious. If one can keep the heart rate variability capacity of the young for a long time in later life one can avoid serious problems like heart attacks. It is shown with the latest technology that the heart rate variability of childhood can be restored in adults by instilling the capacity to love and help others in this world. All negative feelings of the present day world like hatred, jealousy, anger, frustration, loneliness and pride reduce the heart rate variability – the most important protective factor for long and happy life on this planet.

Dr. Ramesh Kapadia, a noted cardiologist of India, has taken the right step in this direction to educate our people in the right methods of healthy life-style. His book gives one the necessary guidance to achieve the right environment for healthy growth and healthful living. Holistic living, with a mind full of love for others, is the best preventive against most, if not all, degenerative disorders. It is better than lowering one's cholesterol or sugar. The methods advocated by Dr. Kapadia are excellent and have been advised even in the Ayurvedic literature. This time-honoured wisdom of the East has to spread to the West as well. I am sure that this book will serve that purpose very well. I wish the book the success that it richly deserves.

Kasturba Medical College,
Mangalore-575 001

B. M. Hegde,
Dean

MD., FRCP (London)., FRCP (Edin).,
FRCP (Glasg)., FACC.,
Visiting Professor of Cardiology,
The Middlesex Hospital Medical School,
University of London.

vi

INTRODUCTION

Coronary Heart Disease remains an enigma so far. Its incidence is increasing even amongst the young all over the world. In India it is alarmingly high. The tell-tale causes of the disease are high blood pressure, diabetes, high serum cholesterol, heredity, smoking, etc.

In treating the coronary disease we have relied almost exclusively on the physically based therapies – drugs, dietary manipulation, exercise, surgical procedures such as bypass surgery and angioplasty. Very valuable as these approaches are we have realised that they are incomplete, frequently ineffective, costly, and sometimes dangerous. Moreover, in many cases of the coronary disease, specially among the young, the tell-tale factors are frequently absent.

The disease being purely a physical event is now being questioned by the modern science. The coronary disease, specially, over and above being physical, has important psychosocial and spiritual aspects. Even the genetically determined disease like diabetes is known to be affected by mental attitudes. The element of human consciousness has once again entered the scene of medicine. The beginning of the 20th century saw a great change in the concepts of physics. The observer's consciousness is considered to be significant in every observation of physics. The new physics is termed as Quantum Physics as against the Classical Physics of Newton.

Now the medical science is also evolving on new lines where the consciousness of the individual is considered to be a very vital factor in the treatment of apparent physical ailments

Some factors, specially an acute sense of isolation along with hostility, self-centredness, cynicism, job and family stresses, are now considered major causes of the rising incidence of the coronary disease amongst the young. This has been relatively a recent observation in understanding the complex problem of the coronary disease. In this book we have attempted to explain how these mental attitudes result in the coronary disease, what is the antidote to these poisons which harm the heart.

Verily the antidote is within the individual himself. How our ancient yogic discipline helps the individual to discover it is explained in this book.

Ahmedabad
2nd Oct. 1995
36, Jain Society
Ellis Bridge,
Ahmedabad -380 006

Ramesh I. Kapadia

THE PUBLISHER'S NOTE

Here is *Heart Disease : A New Direction* by Dr. Ramesh I. Kapadia, the founder of the Universal Healing Program, which has a great positive impact on the management of Coronary Heart Disease. Every year since October 2, 1991, when the Program was launched, the foundation-day is celebrated by the publication of very interesting and instructive books by our distinguished author: *The Primer of Universal Healing* ('92) followed by its Gujarati version ('93) and *Wealth of Food Health of Heart* accompanied by its Gujarati translation ('93). We feel gratified by the overwhelming response of the readers.

The knowledge enables a man to realise that he is The Soul with a body. Now in his ignorance, he thinks that he is a body with a soul.

- *Swami Chinmayanand*

ix

ACKNOWLEDGEMENT

I feel happy to present to the readers my fourth book ever since the inception of the Universal Healing Program four years ago. At the outset I am indebted to my dear participants of the Program. But for them nothing would have been achieved. Yashvantbhai Shukla, Rameshbhai Dave, Jayant Zalavadia, Nandlal Shah, Anilbhai Gandhi have been with us all along. We are grateful to no end to the C. N. Campus and the Trustees. Shri Mahendra Shah, Hon. Sec. of the Trust and his wife Indiraben are a great asset.

The contribution of Janak Acharya, our yoga teacher, Hasumatibehn Vaghani, our dietician, and Dr. Jyotsnaben Patel, our researcher, to the Program is notable. Jitendra Desai of Navajivan Trust has taken a great care of our publications. I must also thank Harivallabh Bhayani for his scholarly suggestions and Vimal Shah, Leelaben Visaria and Narayan Sheth for their help in the analytical research. Govind Mistry and J. D. Trivedi deserve thanks for their assistance. I also appreciate the staff who look after the auditorium.

But for the encouragement and support of my wife Dr. Kokila this book should not have taken shape.

CONTENTS

Foreword v
Introduction vii
Publisher's Note ix
Acknowledgement x

1. Change and Stress 1

2. Nonphysical Causes of CHD 4
    * Isolation
    * Hostility
    * Selfcentredness
    * Cynicism
    * Job Stress
    * Family Stress
    * Greed and Money Function Curve

3. Indepth Stress Management 14

    * Abdominal Breathing
    * Meditation
    * Visualization
    * Auto-Suggestions
    * Ithaka
    * Lessons from Geese
    * Diet and Yoga
    * Sleep and Relaxation Response Compared
    * Stress and Relaxation Response Compared
    * Yin & Yang (Female and Male)

xi

4. Chronic Angina   30

5. Fear of Death   32

6. Author's Letter to Dr. Larry Dossey   33

7. Some Reflections on CHD   38

8. Allopathy and Alternative Therapies   42

9. Experiences Abroad   43

10. Feedbacks   47

11. Tomorrow's Prescription for CHD   53

12. Epilogue   56

Appendices

A   Letter of Dr. Dean Ornish
    to Mrs. Clinton   58
B   Radio Interview   62
C   Universal Healing Program   68
D   Heart Disease Reversal
    Collaborative Net Work   77

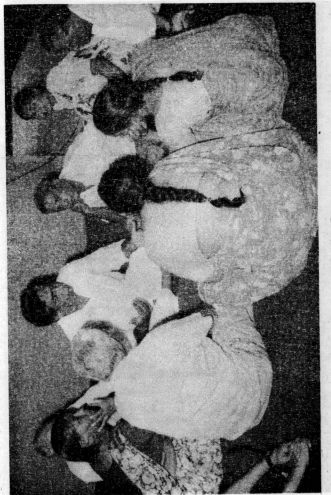

Universal Healing Program

Universal Healing Program

1. CHANGE AND STRESS

Life is in a constant flux, continually changing. Life without change is hard to imagine. Every moment the cells of our body are continually changing; the old ones die and the new ones replace them almost instantaneously. We welcome most of the changes as we grow into youth from boyhood and then into adulthood. We are also happy to see our children growing up into young men and women, and getting happily married and settled. However, there are a number of changes which cause stress, e.g. failure in studies, death of a parent or a dear one, prolonged illness of a member of the family, a serious accident, financial crisis, etc. All the changes have their effect upon the coronary circulation. The coronary arteries respond to the stressful changes with contraction of their muscles resulting in the narrowing of their lumen. The blood circulating in the coronary arteries also becomes thicker in consistency in response to stress. It is now realised that the effect of any stress depends upon its perception by the individual. In other words, what a person makes of that situation is important. The eminent American physician, Dr. Larry Dossey, in his

1

celebrated book *Meaning and Medicine* explains very vividly how the meaning changes physiology of the body. The book starts with a very meaningful quotation of the world-famous physicist, Dr. David Bohm, "Meaning is Being". Our existence depends upon what we make of the various incidents that happen in our day to day life. David Bohm illustrates this with a small anecdote. He had been once to a late night movie show in London with his wife. After the show, he could not start his car, and they were alone in the parking plot. They decided to catch a nearby underground train to go home, and they started walking towards the underground station. It was past mid-night. The road was deserted. There was a fear of getting mugged. They started walking fast towards the station. Suddenly a shadow appeared to follow them. They increased their pace. The shadow also followed with the increasing speed. Now the station was at hand, and they sped faster. They felt their hearts beating fast and their foreheads filled with sweat. Suddenly the shadow came upon them shouting, "David, David, do you need any help?" When they saw that the shadow was of their friend who wanted to help them they felt relieved. Their heartbeats became quieter – a sense of relief came all over them. What a stark difference it makes to the body by mere interpretation of the shadow! If you interpret the shadow as your friend, the response is quite different from one when you interpret it as your enemy.

In the days of Newton and Descartes the body and the mind were considered distinctly separate. The end of the 19th century saw the rise of psychosomatic medicine, and it began to be realised that the mind and the body are intimately connected with each other. And that the mind can effect great changes in the body was proved by the development of biofeedback and auto-suggestions therapy in many diseases. Now with the development of science the role of consciousness affecting not only the individual body but also everything that exists in the universe has come to light. The mind is now understood as not something present in the brain only but also in all the cells of the body all over and even beyond.

2. NONPHYSICAL CAUSES OF CHD

Isolation

Isolation is a major cause of coronary heart disease, skin diseases, and even cancer. Isolation is not merely loneliness or solitude. It is a sense of aloofness, unconnectedness, even alienation. It is an emotional condition, an acute feeling that a person is left all alone high and dry in almost all situations that matter to him or have a meaning of his existence. Often retirement leads to this condition. For instance, a retired executive, who has enjoyed power once, feels that now that he is out of office people have ceased to respect him. A young man striving to build his career may have a stern boss or uncooperative and hostile colleagues to deal with; and is compelled to continue in his job suppressing his anger and helplessness. A talented person might feel that his talent is not recognised, he is not appreciated and feels quite bitter. Even domestic discord and tension might make one feel rather isolated in one's home in the midst of near and dear ones. A spouse might feel isolated when one of the couple feels neglected by the other who might be over-occupied and lost in his or her pursuits. A child might feel isolated when parents are too busy to give due attention and care, particularly if the child has a problem and needs support. Loss of a spouse after a long and happy married life creates a void and is a major risk-factor resulting in heart attack or even cancer during the first year of bereavement. At times a virtuous person laments the lack of virtue all around and might feel isolated. Metaphysical anguish also causes isolation. In short, the causes of isolation are numerous and complex. In the modern world of wholesale competition, stress and isolation creep in from all directions. Isolation is spiritual when a person drifts away from his inner self and pursues job, business and social commitments quite against his conscience. Isolation often breeds hostility, cynicism, selfcentredness, a sense of guilt and gloom which lead to serious illness, particularly coronary heart disease. It has a very adverse effect on the body, specially on the immune system and blood chemistry. The isolated individual may take to alcohol, tobacco-chewing, and smoking which might further aggravate the risk of coronary heart disease. When a person feels that he alone is pitchforked in a particular situation or predicament, he feels isolated like that Hunchback of Notre Dame or one struck with leprosy or leucoderma. When one is irrascible, frustrated, gloomy or over egocentric he is isolated.

How to overcome isolation? The way is to connect. But then how do we connect? We have a very heartening evidence of experience of our universal healing program. Meditation does heal isolation. Our major limitation is that we perceive ourselves limited to space and time. In our non-meditative mood our mind keeps on wandering from the present moment back into the past and forth into the future and thus uprooting us from the present; this isolates us. During meditation one cultivates the habit of staying in the present moment – the eternal NOW. And being one with the breath, which is *prana* or life-force, is to experience the state of being connected with one's larger self and through that with the whole universe. This ultimately results in peace and calm of mind reflected in the increase in the alpha activity of the brain. In other words, to meditate is to connect; and the moment one gets connected isolation ebbs away.

Along with meditation, group discussion and the sharing of feeling are also effective means of freedom from isolation. After meditation one feels at peace with not only one's own self but also with the world at large. This encourages the individual to share feeling through group discussion. This is also a vital aspect of our healing program. It has a magic effect of relieving isolation. During group discussion, through heart-to-heart exchange of ideas, which might not necessarily solve a problem, the load of the pent up feeling of isolation is taken off and one experiences great relief.

Isolation is painful because it saps the real joy of living. It distances us from the inner sources of joy, peace, and strength. It is a great drain on one's potential as a human being. In the treatment of isolation there is a need to connect with the world within (vertical connection) and the world without (horizontal connection).

Hostility

The dictionary meaning of hostility is 'revengeful attitude'. In its larger sense it includes extreme intolerance, aggressive behaviour, unreasonable anger and dislike for an individual. Normally we consider tolerance as a virtue, but in reality if you tolerate halfheartedly with an inner dislike, it is nothing but the suppressed anger, and it has the same deleterious effect as anger has on the heart. Hostility can be due to the lack of parental care during childhood which results in a sense of insecurity and injustice at home or at school from colleagues and teachers. Children who have experienced such injustice during childhood feel very bitter about everything, and develop hostility against the whole world on slightest pretext. Hostility breeds extremely irritable temper and selfcentredness with cynical attitude towards everything. With this temperament one looks at everyone with contempt and feels isolated.

Test Your Hostility Level

To get an impression of how hostile you tend to be, answer the following questions in each of the 3 areas that research has shown to be critical: cynicism, anger, and aggression. Though this questionnaire is not a scientifically validated test; it will give you a sense of how you measure in these 3 aspects of hostility.

Cynicism

☐ When in the express lane at the supermarket, do you often count the number of items in the baskets of the people in front of you to make sure that they are not over the limit?

☐ When an elevator does not come as quickly as you think it should, do your thoughts focus on the inconsiderate behaviour of the person on another floor who is holding it up?

☐ Do you frequently check up on family members or coworkers to make sure that they have not committed a mistake in a certain task?

Anger

☐ When you are held up in a slow line of traffic, the bank, or the supermarket, do you feel your heart pounding and your breath quickening?

☐ When minor things go wrong, do you feel like lashing out at the world?

☐ When someone criticizes you, do you begin to feel annoyed?

Aggression

☐ If an elevator stops too long on the floor above you, are you likely to pound on the door?

☐ If people mistreat you, do you look for an opportunity to pay them back, just for the principle of the matter?

☐ Do you frequently find yourself muttering at the TV during a news broadcast?

If you have answered yes to at least one question in each section or to four or more questions overall, then your hostility level is probably high.

This questionnaire was taken from page 79 of the book *Mind Body Medicine* by Daniel Goleman, Ph.D.

Selfcentredness

Selfcentredness arises out of a sense of utter insecurity. When an individual feels very insecure, he seeks self-interest without the least concern for others. Even at the prospect of harming others he sticks to self-interest. One becomes so very egocentric that it tends to narrow not only one's outlook on life but also one's arteries.

Cynicism

When an individual finds fault with everything, good or bad, and has lost all faith in goodness of life, he becomes contemptuously cynical; and this attitude again, according to Dr. Dean Ornish, poisons the heart.

Job Stress

Stress due to the insecurity of job, a sense of injustice, a constant tussle with the boss, non-cooperation of colleagues, ambition to rise above everyone else in a short time, jealousy and vicious competition are the apparent causes of heart attack amongst the young. In business, financial, managerial and labour problems cause great stress.

A 35-year old young employee of the State Bank of India, who had come under the influence of Sri Aurobindo and Mataji was living a contented healthy life. At one of the exams conducted by the Bank for promotion, a colleague with much less competence got the promotion and he was left out. For nearly three years he remained stressed under the sense of severe injustice and felt isolated. He was struck with a coronary episode. After angiography he was even advised bypass surgery. A great sense of dissatisfaction and alienation from the whole world probably resulted in coronary heart disease.

Family Stress

An unexpected financial crisis, a long drawn expensive illness, marital problems, shocking catastrophic family events and conflicts with children are usually the causes of the family stress which may also result in coronary heart disease in the individuals who are prone to it on other scores.

10

Greed

We live in a socioeconomic set-up where for the whole day one has to work hard at the inhuman speed of physical and intellectual work. Man has come to believe that to move physically and intellectually is to live. The way we move we go on collecting things at material level, knowledge on the intellectual level, and experience on the sensual and physical level. With every experience and achievement, we build up our ego and create an enclosure around us. In that enclosure we feel secure and live secluded and isolated from our real self because of the sense of possession.

Greed is a very common human trait. If something benefits an individual he would naturally like to have more of it. In pursuit of anything whether it is name, fame, money, possessing rare antique articles, books, paintings, and other worldly goods there is a thin line between greed and ambition. Even in good pursuits like spreading humanitarian ideas, such as usefulness of yoga in everyday life, one may overstep.

Money Function Curve

The accompanying money function curve demonstrates how greed for material possessions is self-defeating in the end. The Money Function Curve shows the amount of money spent and the fulfilment that money brings. First, the amount of money spent is for survival. The amount of money spent increases to bring you to a level of comfort. The amount of money spent then brings you to a level of luxury. Once the amount of money spent goes beyond the point of luxury, you begin purchasing your own death in instalments. As the function curve shows, the individual begins to experience irritability, death of "feeling brain", insomnia, social and legal problems, and diseases.

MONEY FUNCTION CURVE

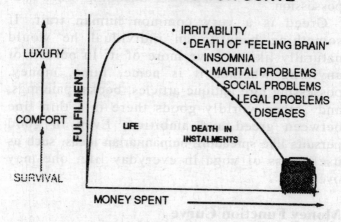

Courtesy : © 1993 Naras Bhat M.D; Stress Cybernetix

12

"Every affection of the mind that is attended with pain or pleasure, hope or fear, is the cause of an agitation, whose influence extends to the heart." This golden quotation of William Harvey summarises succinctly the effects of emotions on the heart. Coronary arteries are very sensitive to emotions, good or bad. The intensity of emotion results in the narrowing of the coronary artery and increased viscosity of blood. We have seen that psychosocial factors like hostility, selfcentredness, cynicism, isolation along with family and job stress are the major causes of the rising incidence of coronary heart disease. It is obvious that the routine medical management including drugs and surgery is not able to deal with these root causes of the problem. Psychotherapy and psychotropic drugs also help marginally in mitigating the effects of these factors and that too, not without some undesirable side effects. On the other hand the indepth stress management on the lines of the Universal Healing Program has proved its usefulness in a big way.

The man who gets angry at the right things and with right people and in the right way and at the right time and for the right length of time is commended.

- Aristotle

3. INDEPTH STRESS MANAGEMENT

The indepth stress management of coronary heart disease is now a vital part of the total management of coronary heart disease. Recognition of stress as a cause of heart disease is not new. However, the approach to stress in recent years has taken a new shape. Until now stress was managed by psychotherapy and tranquillizers. Now the patient himself is taught to manage stress.

The landmark work of Dr. Dean Ornish based on the ancient yogic Indian traditions has opened up new vistas in the management of coronary heart disease.

Abdominal Breathing

The abdominal breathing now enjoys prominent position in stress management. In adult life breathing is largely thoracic and at times abdominal. The practice of abdominal breathing is almost forgotten by the time we grow out of childhood. An infant breathes only abdominally. Of late the advantages of abdominal breathing have been understood very clearly. It at once calms the sympathetic system and activates parasympathetic system, reducing the heart rate, systolic blood pressure, oxygen requirement of the heart and the viscosity of blood. In short, it acts like beta-blokers without any side effects. The abdominal breathing requires some practice. However, it is very simple and easy to practise in almost any situation. Once the technique is mastered, one may practise it daily, at least 3-4 times a day, for 10-15 breaths each time. The benefits derived from abdominal breathing may diminish if you are not regular in your practice. The effect of this yogic exercise is also dose-related. We call it 'Yogic Exercise' because it is a very useful tool for getting mental and physical relaxation. When an individual practises meditation, the mind becomes quieter with the abdominal breathing; the peace of mind that follows has a great power to heal. Healing follows the production of alpha activity in the brain and secretion of endorphins and health giving immunoglobins. Above all an individual experiences oneness with his larger Self within. This connects him with the wide world. Our participants who have regularly practised meditation and abdominal breathing have experienced a sense of great empowerment in their daily activities. Some have admitted to have gained greater control over their temper. Some have observed that they were able to modify their taste for fried foods and sweets without feeling deprived of them. They experience greater power over their life through this yogic practice.

Abdominal breathing is a powerful tool to bring about relaxation and activate the right brain. Only a minute of abdominal breathing with awareness kept on the inhalation and exhalation brings about the *Yin* mode of existence with all its benefits. The relaxation response is superior to the relaxation achieved during sleep.

Meditation

Meditation is beginning to occupy a place in the conventional treatment of coronary heart disease. It has come to stay as an essential part of management along with medication and surgery. The stress management which was done uptil now with the help of psychotherapy, tranquillizers and group support now includes meditation in its therapeutic armamentarium.

Meditation is simply being in the present moment. The present moment frees the individual to change, explore new patterns, pleasures, and possibilities. It is a powerful way to heal isolation. The sense of isolation has been incriminated as the single most important factor in the rising incidence of coronary heart disease amongst the young who are prone to it on other scores (heredity, hypercholesteroloemia, diabetes, etc.)

There are many ways to meditate. No one way is best for everyone. One thing common to all forms of meditation is the art of paying attention. We do a lot of different things at the same time.

In order to meditate first pay attention to breathing. Breathing is central to every aspect of meditation training. It is a wonderful place to focus the mind. Breath is a rich experience. It connects us with the whole universe. When you try to pay attention to breathing, you notice that the mind starts wandering. The wandering of the mind is a normal state of mind. From the meditative perspective the normal state of mind is severely suboptimal. It is more asleep than awake. Its energy is frittered away in thoughts of past and future. It is rarely in the present moment. Human beings have a capacity of shifting their awareness wherever they wish. Normally, individuals who have not been trained to meditate keep their awareness on the mind which has the habit of wandering. Cultivating and developing a capacity to keep the awareness in the present moment instead of the wandering mind is all what meditation is about. When you start focussing your awareness on breathing, you begin to ride the waves of breath, in and out. At this moment, the awareness begins to wander to the thoughts. Willingly, gently and kindly bring it back to the breath. If it wanders a million times, just lasso it back to breath a million times. This will train the mind to settle at one place. When the mind is thus cultivated, you begin to feel that you are in the present moment – time slows down and might even seem to stop. You are in a NOW, that is, continually unfolding. The moment you are in touch with the present moment, almost everything

17

will become more vivid and alive. The calm experienced in meditation brings about penetrative insight (into our experience in the present moment). From this insight comes greater understanding, and therefore greater freedom to conduct our lives. The way we feel would lead to greater wisdom and happiness. The deep physiological relaxation which occurs in meditation is in itself healing. There is an access to deep inner resources for healing, the mind operating more effectively and helping to develop strategies, making sensible adaptive choices under pressure while coping with stress. One feels more engaged in life.

Meditation is a way of living which introduces us to that other part of our consciousness which is the common ground of all humanity. There we are not individuals; we are not separate entities with psychological content; where each one of us is actually the rest of humanity. As Guru of Dalai Lama explained, "anger, jealousy, hatred and aggression" thrive on concept of our inherent separate existence. Now all the recent researches in physics reveal that our separate existence is an illusion even if it is a stubborn one. In meditation we experience the emptiness of the concept of separate existence. This frees us from the qualities that separate us, and it generates in us compassion, love, and altruism which unite us.

Visualization

Visualization is an imaginative process of forming pictures in the mind's eye. When we visualize in a non-meditative mood, i.e. when our mind is full of other thoughts, visualization is not effective because it is unfocussed and passive. However, during meditation, visualization becomes active and focussed. Like the sunrays converging through a magnifying glass burn the paper, visualization during meditation brings about the desired effects. In our Program the participants visualize in a variety of ways : how their coronary circulation and function of heart improve and how they feel energetic in their daily routine. The beauty of this visualization is that though there may be no anatomical or physiological relevance to their imagination, even then it improves the clinical condition of the patient. Dr. Dean Ornish has also noted it to be useful to his participants.

Visualization also includes forgiving an individual who has done a great wrong or injustice to you in the past. This is a very difficult task. However, the participant is taught to condone not so much the act which was obviously wrong and unjust; he is asked to bring in front of his mind's eye the image of the person who perpetrated the wrong and believe that the individual was ignorant and childish in his behaviour and hence he be pardoned for his irresponsible act. Thus the practitioner of visualization becomes free from the feeling of hostility against that individual. In other words, the thought of that individual loses the power to hurt him. Similarly, if the person himself is suffering from a sense of guilt, having done some wrong in the past, he may bring his own picture before the mind's eye and forgive self for the thoughtless act. This does not necessarily mean that he absolves himself from the responsibility of the wrong deed. Thus he releases himself from the feeling of guilt which keeps on haunting him. After getting freedom from the sense of guilt he may resolve not to behave in such a manner again in future. So, the whole exercise of visualization during meditation is a very powerful weapon to heal the deep-rooted isolation. A participant in Dr. Dean Ornish's program, who was a retired army officer, said that the act of forgiving through visualization is more powerful than the most powerful weapons he ever used in the army.

Auto-suggestions

During the relaxed state of the body and the mind (Shavasana) our participants are taught to use auto-suggestions to improve coronary circulation.

Auto-suggestions during meditation also have a very powerful effect on the physiology of the body. This has been the subject of bio-feedback and self-hypnosis in the management of various illnesses. We have taken help of auto-suggestions in our Program for even changing the food habits.

The beneficial effect of auto-suggestions in choosing the food habit of the participant is a subject of active research. Auto-suggestions during meditation increase the inner strength of an individual to choose the right type of food and enjoy it and feel empowered to give up eating his most favourite dishes. He can let go his favourite dairy-rich chocolate ice-cream without feeling the sense of deprivation and experience the fact that he can now do without it.

ITHAKA

[Ithaka is an island off the western coast of Greece, the native place of Odyssus, who travelled across the lands and seas after the fall of Troy. He met with many hazards and miracles in his voyage on his way to Ithaka.]

In this poem Ithaka is a metaphor for the land of our heart's desire. In quest of one's dreamland one encounters many difficulties as well as adventures. But with courage one must sail on. It is this journey which is important; travelling is more important than arriving. While travelling one enjoys seeing the world around, living in the present moment.

When you ultimately reach your Ithaka and perhaps find it not so fascinating as in your dreams, do not despair. Your experience during travelling has so much enriched you that you will understand what Ithakas mean!

ITHAKA

As you set out for Ithaka
hope your road is a lone one,
full of adventure, full of discovery.
Laistrygonians, Cyclops,
angry Posiedon – don't be afraid of them:
you'll never find things like that on your way
as long as a rare excitement
stirs your spirit and your body.
Laistrygonians, Cyclops,
wild Poseidon – you won't encounter them
unless you bring them along inside your soul,
unless your soul sets them up in front of you.

Hope that your road is a long one.
May there be many summer mornings when,
with what pleasure, what joy,
you enter harbors you're seeing for the first
        time;
may you stop at Phoenician trading stations
to buy fine things,
mother of pearl and coral, amber and ebony,
sensual perfume of every kind –
as many sensual perfumes as you can;
and may you visit many Egyptian cities
to learn and go on learning from their scholars.

Keep Ithaka always in your mind.
Arriving there is what you're destined for.
But don't hurry the journey at all.
Better if it lasts for years,

so you're old by the time you reach the island,
wealthy with all you've gained on the way,
not expecting Ithaka to make you rich.

Ithaka gave you the marvelous journey.
Without her you wouldn't have set out.
She has nothing left to give you now.

And if you find her poor, Ithaka won't have
fooled you.
Wise as you will have become, so full of
experience,
you'll have understood by then what these
Ithakas mean.

– C. P. Cavafy

Lessons From Geese
by
Milton Olson

1. As each bird flaps its wings, it creates an "uplift" for the bird following. By flying in a "V" formation, the whole flock adds 71% greater flying range than if the bird flew alone.

Lesson: People who share common direction and sense of community can get where they are going quicker and easier because they are travelling on the thrust of one another.

2. Whenever a goose falls out of formation, it suddenly feels the drag and resistance of trying to fly alone, and quickly gets back into formation to take advantage of the "lifting power" of the bird immediately in front.

Lesson : If we have as much sense as a goose, we will stay in formation with those who are headed where we want to go (and be willing to accept their help as well as give ours to the others).

3. When the lead goose gets tired, it rotates back into the formation and another goose flies at the point position.

Lesson : It pays to take turns doing the hard tasks and sharing leadership – with people, as with geese, we are interdependent on each other.

4. The geese in formation honk from behind to encourage those up front to keep up their speed.

Lesson : We need to make sure our honking from behind is encouraging – and not something else.

5. When a goose gets sick or wounded or shot down, two geese drop out of formation and follow it down to help and protect it. They stay with it until it is able to fly again or dies. Then they launch out on their own, with another formation, or catch up with the flock.

Lesson : If we have as much sense as geese, we too will stand by each other in difficult times as well as when we are strong.

Diet and Yoga

We have already published a book entitled *Wealth of Food, Health of Heart*. A mention about diet in the present context is due to our realization that diet is intimately connected with the successful yogic exercises like abdominal breathing, *shavasana* and meditation. The practice of these yogic disciplines promotes the motivation of the participants to take a low fat vegetarian diet. The intake of low fat vegetarian diet makes the yogic practices of meditation and *shavasana* easier for the participants. Diet and yogic exercises complement each other.

Sleep and Relaxation Response Compared

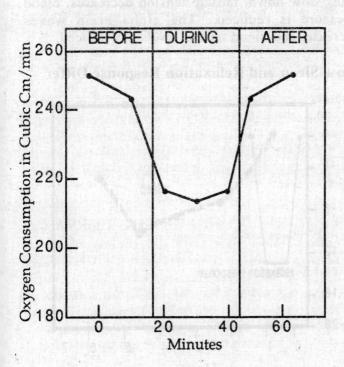

25

How Metabolism Changes with the Relaxation Response :

The body's metabolic rate that measures the overall biochemical activity is reflected in the amount of oxygen consumed. This graph shows that oxygen consumption is reduced significantly in the meditators when they switch from resting (before) on to meditating (during) and again rises once meditation is stopped (after).

In the relaxation response, respiration and heart rates slow down, muscle tension decreases, blood pressure is reduced. The alpha brain waves increase, and blood lactate levels are reduced.

How Sleep and Relaxation Response Differ

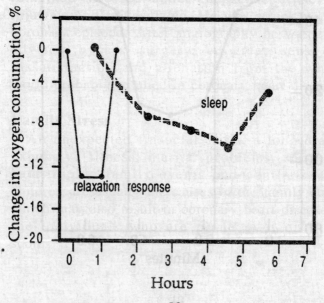

Though sleep and the relaxation response both cause a decrease in oxygen consumption, there is a much more significant decrease in the relaxation response. Though the graph only shows the relaxation response for a short amount of time this decrease will remain for as long as the relaxation response is elicited.

Reference: Benson, Herbert, and Klipper; *The Relaxation Response.* New York: Avon, 1976

Stress and Relaxation Response Compared

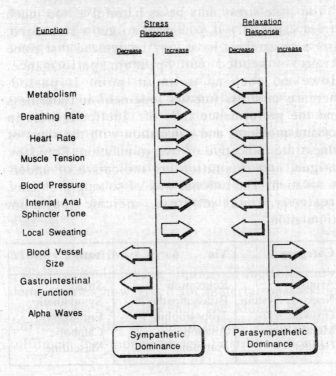

The above (see page 34) chart shows how sympathetic dominance leads to wear and tear, and para-sympathetic dominance promotes healing.

Yin - Yang

According to Chinese philosophy we human beings perform throughout our life either in Yin mode or Yang mode. Balance of both is required for happy and meaningful existence. Yin characterises a relaxation response and Yang stress response.

Too little stress may be as harmful as too much stress especially if you want to get a task done. Stress researchers have long recognized that some stress is needed for optimum performance. However, once an optimum point is passed, increase in stress impairs judgment and alertness and the performance falls off. Ineffectiveness in solving problems and exhaustion with the signs of illness are indicative of overstimulation. Boredom, fatigue, and frustration are indicative of understimulation. The rational way of solving problems, creativity, and progress indicate optimum stimulation.

Category	Yin	Yang
Arousal	Relaxation	Stress
Nervous System	Parasympathetic	Sympathetic
Growth	Tropotrophic	Ergotrophic
Metabolism	Anabolic	Catabolic
Gender	Feminine	Masculine

Category	Yin	Yang
Activity	Receptive	Active
Subjectivity	Subjective	Objective
Experience	Experiential	Experimental, Empirical
Brainside	Right Brain	Left Brain
Consciousness	Transcendental	Agitated
	Sleep	Awake
Brainwaves	Alpha, Theta, Delta	Beta
Attitude	Intuitive	Analytical
	Sacred	Secular
	Spiritual	Science, Materialism
	Mystery	Mastery
	Human Being	Human Doing
	Wholeness	Parts
	Quality	Quantity
Rhythm	Melody	Notes
Separation	Synthetic	Analytical
	Process	Form
	Expansion	Contraction
Dependence	Interdependent	Independent
	Adapt, Co-operate	Confront, Fight
	Connected	Lonely
Emotion	Love	Hostility
Chemistry	Alkaline	Acid
Nutrition	Nourishment	Nutrients

4. CHRONIC ANGINA

Chronic stable angina is a fairly common manifestation of the coronary disease. Most patients with chronic angina can lead a very useful life with the help of the nitrate group of drugs. Angina is chronic when it occurs after a particular mental or physical stress or a heavy meal and is relieved instantly with some rest or a nitrate pill under the tongue. Such angina is rarely fatal. Only in a few cases chronic angina is so severe that it may require treatment with angioplasty or bypass surgery.

More than 200 years ago Dr. John Hunter, a very famous British surgeon, suffered from chronic angina. At that time nitrate was available in a capsule form, to be broken in a handkerchief and its vapour inhaled through the nose to relieve the chest pain. John Hunter lived a very busy life with angina for 40 years. One day he was requested by the superintendent of a hospital to be present at an interview where a lady doctor was to be selected for the post of Obstetrician and Gynaecologist. Looking through the files of the applicants, one of the candidates was found most deserving for the post. The Superintendent along with Dr. Hunter and another colleague decided to select that person. In course of the interview somebody brought in a small note for the Superintendent which he read and slipped quietly into his pocket. When all the interviews were over and a decision was to be taken, the Superintendent, who was also the chairperson, suddenly changed the decision. Seeing that he was influenced by that note, Dr. Hunter burst out in great anger, and throwing the file on the floor dashed out of the board room and dropped dead outside. During his lifetime Dr. John Hunter used to say, "My life is in the hands of the hooligans who choose to irritate me. When I die, you should look at my heart; the arteries supplying blood to my heart would have hardened like a rock."

Dr. Hunter's wish was honoured. On examining his heart after his death, it was seen that the arteries had hardened. Hunter's heart is preserved in the Royal College of Surgeon Museum at London and below it is the inscription relating the above story. The story has two lessons. Chronic angina is compatible with a long useful existence, and a sudden burst of emotion, specially anger, can be a death-blow to the heart.

5. FEAR OF DEATH

Coronary Heart Disease is notorious for killing the victim in an instant. Angina occurring for the first time, angina at rest, and the frequent episodes of angina not responding satisfactorily to nitrates require intensive medical, and if necessary even surgical treatment. However, the fear of death with every episode of angina is out of the place. Fear leads to the narrowing of the coronary arteries and increase in viscosity of blood which may aggravate angina. Longer the standing of chronic angina, the greater is the establishment of collateral circulation. Moreover, in the patients of chronic angina the heart muscle gets conditioned to ischoemia.

A clinical assessment of angina in a given individual is a very complex problem which requires consideration of several factors – age, sex, family history, personal habits like smoking, alcohol and regularity in taking prescribed medicines, etc. The decision regarding the management has to be highly individualised. No general rule of the thumb is possible. Moreover, a final word is not yet written on the management of coronary heart disease and the differences of opinion amongst the experts are common. Doctor-patient relationship and faith in the doctor play an important role.

6. AUTHOR'S LETTER TO
DR. LARRY DOSSEY

This communication throws light on the views
of the author on the problem of CHD.

24 Dec., 1992

My dear Larry,

Thank you very much for your loving letter of
November 11, 1992. I was overwhelmed by your
generous estimate of our modest effort of *Primer
of Universal Healing*. This brings to you and
Barbara our cart-load of best wishes for Xmas
and New Year.

Ever since 1958, the days of my post-graduate
training in UK, enigmatic coronary heart disease
has fascinated me. I have been very fortunate to
study it in a vast variety of individuals – quite a
few during acute episode of myocardial infarction
and a formidable follow-up of patients with stable
ischoemic heart disease. The disease has earned
notoriety of being highly unpredictable. It is my
experience that a lot depends on the attitude of
the patient and his attending physician towards the

33

disease rather than on the actual extent of the disease. The variable element, spasm in an atherosclerotic coronary artery and increased viscosity of blood are greater culprits than the fixed narrowing of the coronary arteries due to atherosclerosis. The fixed lesions are probably responsible for chronic stable disease which is rarely fatal. When the symptoms due to the chronic stable disease are disabling, preventing patient from enjoying normal life, surgical intervention may become necessary. Nevertheless, it is observed that in a large number of patients adequate drug therapy assisted by attention to hygienic details such as low fat vegetarian diet, weight control, about 40 minute walk daily and in-depth stress management with progressive deep relaxation, meditation, and the sharing of feeling through group discussion bring about amazingly good results. Particularly, meditation motivates healthy life-style changes. In some cases even the reversal of atherosclerotic changes has also been noted. Very encouraging results of this approach in case of patients with severe CHD are most heartening. In the treatment of acute myocardial infarction, the crucial factor, it seems to me, is the reassuring capacity and confidence of the attending physician.

Larry, I certainly do not underrate the value of intensive care monitoring and investigations such as computerized treadmill test, 2 D Echo studies, scanning (Thallium, PET, etc.), coronary angiography and palliative procedures like angioplasty, CABG, and even cardiomyplasty when LV function is severely compromised. However, in a large majority of CHD patients a cost effective simple approach of judicious use of drugs along with hygienic measures by a skilled physician well versed in art and science of medicine is all that is required. That will prove far more fruitful than the routine run of the mill approach which might be forbiddingly expensive and yet not quite effective.

A very vexed and intriguing aspect of CHD is the sudden death due to acute myocardial infarction. This is not always related to the extent of infarcted area but it is due to sudden occurrence of ventricular fibrillation due to acute ischoemia. It is probably due to the response of the whole individual to acute ischoemic insult. I have a feeling that the incidence of sudden death may also diminish in the wake of altered healthier response to the stress of ischoemia by in-depth stress management.

Almost all the participants of our program within a matter of six to eight weeks admit to a changed attitude of confidence as against the fear of sudden death. Their outlook towards life circumstances, family as well as work-life becomes healthier and their world-view becomes one of cooperation and compassion as against competition and survival.

Conviction about effectiveness of this approach occurred to me fourteen years ago when I read my paper on "Rehabilitation after Myocardial Infarction" at the International meet held in Bombay in 1978.

Larry, allow me to extend a bit my rambling: utter selfishness, greed, hatred, vicious rivalries, terrorism, drug addiction! Are not these ills stemming from a sense of isolation, a false sense of ego and the lack of real identity? The precious human existence is frittered away in petty squabbles and misdirected ambitions and goals. With extraordinary technological leaps and all-round information and communication explosion, it is natural to be carried off one's feet unless one's inner moorings are firmly set on the rock of the belief that love, compassion, and altruism are the only attributes which distinguish the human from the animal. Without these human attributes all the treasures of world pale into insignificance. They become a liability instead of an asset. Quiet comforting is the evidence that the human attributes blossom forth as the individual experiences an infinite dimension to his temporal existence during meditation, hence my prescription of simple technique of *shavasana* and meditation for the ills of mankind. Such are my ruminations while pursuing my efforts to tackle the problem of CHD. These thoughts have taken hold of me during all my waking moments. I have shared them with you.

I wonder whether such thoughts should not be published in our reputed medical journals. I feel, it is time physicians with similar thinking came forward to voice their feelings for a cardiac problem of such magnitude and importance in a year of "Heart-beat – The Rhythm of Life" celebrated by WHO.

With most affectionate regards,

Yours very lovingly,

Dr. Ramesh I. Kapadia

With such a vegetarian diet they will live a peaceful and healthy life till ripe old age, and pass on the heritage of such a life to their children.

- Socrates

7. SOME REFLECTIONS ON CORONARY HEART DISEASE

The sudden death which occurs in Coronary Heart Disease has spread its mantle of fear over the whole complex problem of Coronary Heart Disease. However, it needs emphasis that a large number of Coronary Heart Disease patients even after the attack live a meaningful life for a long time. Simple linear mathematical relationships govern most of our thinking in medicine. The dynamic human body does not follow these linear relationships, and doctors tend to predict the unpredictable!

The narrowing of the coronary arteries *per se* does not inevitably result in heart attack. The narrowing of the coronary arteries gradually progresses to a complete block with the passage of time. However, occluded vessel does not pose the risk of a heart attack and its complications or even of a long term detrimental effect on heart function. The complete occlusion resulting in heart attack is almost always the result of a blood clot causing obstruction of a near normal vessel. In the absence of a heart attack, the narrowed coronary artery does not alter the long term changes in the total left ventricular function despite evidence of the exercise induced signs and symptoms of myocardial ischoemia. It has been shown in some brilliant scientific studies that brief periods of ischaemia (so called silent ischaemia) trigger adaptive changes in the heart, protecting it from the future major failure of blood supply. This is called ischaemic preconditioning. In this way silent ischaemia may even prove beneficial to the heart.

No study has shown that the coronary angiography is required as a 'gold standard' test in the diagnosis of Coronary Heart Disease before giving the patient medical therapy. On the contrary, the randomised trials have demonstrated that nitrates, aspirin, low fat vegetarian diet, beta-blockers, calcium-blockers and angiotensin converting enzyme inhibitors can save many lives. The Coronary Artery Surgery Study (CASS) of U.S.A. clearly shows that angiography should be done only to plan the operation after the decision to operate is taken and not as the basis of diagnosis. If angiography is done before that decision, there is a risk of the patient being scared by the doctors that he is sitting on a 'volcano' which may kill him at any time.

For a large number of patients undergoing bypass surgery there is no evidence that it improves their prognosis compared to those managed by medical means. Disturbed coronary anatomy except for the left main artery disease does not predict prognosis when the left ventricular function is good. Even when those with left main artery disease who declined the surgery and were followed up for over a decade, the annual mortality was only 1.3% which is not significantly higher than that of the general population and it was 0% for single and double vessel disease. When obstructed internally coronary arteries are capable of remodelling themselves and enlarging at the site of obstruction. This puts us in mind of our father of medicine, Hippocratis's observation that the body has inherent capacity to heal itself.

In the patients who run the risk of sudden death as a result of the coronary artery disease bypass surgery by and large does not afford any protection. Even the usual claim of better quality of life after the bypass needs appraisal as new thoughts on the quality of life demand more critical appraisal of how it is measured. For angioplasty the restenosis rate may be as high as 50% which is due to the increased cellular and fibrous growth (fibrocellular intimal hyperplasia) for which there is no easy solution in sight.

In conclusion, one definite indication for revascularisation is intractable (not responding to medical therapy) chest pain and another where there is poor left ventricular function with anatomic changes such as aneurysm, ventricular septal defects or mitral leaks, making life miserable for the patients. The coronary bypass surgery is a boon to these very ill patients. We should encourage revascularisation based on the patient's symptoms and disabilities rather than on angiograms with so called critical narrowing of coronary arteries.

All too frequently requested angiograms and advice for angioplasty and bypass surgery by the well intentioned highly qualified doctors is due to a different perception of the disease and its probable outcome in a particular patient. There is indeed a need for rethinking in this field.*

* Doctors as well as the lay readers are requested to see the article by Dr. B. M. Hegde, Kasturba Medical College, Mangalore, India, published in the *Proceedings of the Royal College of Physicians of Edinburg,* July 1995, Volume 25 , Number 3, pages 421-424. The title of the article is : "The Management of Coronary Artery Disease : A Time for Reappraisal".

8. ALLOPATHY
AND
ALTERNATIVE THERAPIES

A time has come for a rational view regarding the usefulness of alternative therapies in treatment of all diseases, specially in those which are not yet amenable to cure by allopathy. An alternative therapy may prove useful in a particular individual for a particular ailment when allopathy fails to help that individual. It is important to keep in mind the tremendous progress done by allopathy in the recent years in eradication of infectious diseases specially tuberculosis and the deadly and disfiguring disease like smallpox. Surgery has also become very safe with the advancement of allopathy. Like any other powerful weapon, the use of which can be either for good or for bad, the indiscriminate use of powerful allopathic drugs may at times harm an individual. This has increased the responsibility of allopathic practitioners. It explains a very intensive curriculum for the graduate and post-graduate students of allopathy. Generally speaking all systems of therapy have some special merits as well as limitations in each of them.

In the evolving medicine of the future any therapeutic approach to be complete will have to treat the body, mind and the soul of the individual.

9. EXPERIENCES ABROAD

Ever since 1991 when I first met Dr. Dean Ornish in California, I have quite closely followed philosophy and practice in the treatment of the Coronary Heart Disease. Almost every year so far I have made it a point to go to the USA in summer to be in the mainstream of the new experimentation. Every trip, I must say, has left me richer and more equipped in my endeavour. I have a host of memories to share.

I had a privilege to be invited on 7th June 1994 to deliver a lecture on 'Universal Healing' at Duke University Medical Centre, N.C., USA to commemorate Dr. Kempner's address to American Medical Association 50 years ago in 1944 on his successful treatment of 50 congestive cardiac failure patients by the "Rice Diet" therapy. Dr. Kempner will be 93 this year. My talk centred round our experience with meditation in healing, meditation being the vital part of universal healing program. At the end of my talk, an old lady in her 80s sprang up on her feet and said : "Doctor, please tell me what is the longevity span today ? I hope to live for 125 years. How could meditation help me?" Almost intuitively I replied, "Mrs. Williams, the way we experience this very moment, peace and joy of the human existence in a climate most congenial such as this, is in itself an everlasting moment, an eternal Now. Is this not enough ? In meditation it is the same awareness, the same experience. The question of dying does not arise at all." "Where shall I learn meditation?" she asked. "Perhaps my books and cassettes might be useful. We are together always. No matter how very apart we be physically."

An encounter with Dr. Dean Ornish's patient is quite memorable. A patient aged 72, who was advised bypass surgery but instead chose to join Dr. Ornish's program was benefited but not to the extent the other participants were. He complained to Dean that he did exactly what others were also doing -- he was a vegetarian and teatotaller and also practised yoga and meditation besides helping the needy. Dean listened to him attentively and said, "Please go ahead in the same way. Don't be burdened by the idea of altruism. Don't be obsessed. Thank God that you have been able to help others and that you are in a fortunate position to do so. Thank even those helped by you. Try this for about eight weeks." The patient got the message of Dean's remarks. Believe it or not, within less than six weeks his angina disappeared. Even the attitude of altruism when loaded with ego is counterproductive.

Some years ago Dr. Larry Dossey studied the speeches of 30 patients for about 15 minutes. He made frequency count of the use of the words "I", "My" or "Mine" in the course of utterance of each one of them. He followed up these individuals for 15 years. To his great surprise, those who had used the word "I", "My" or "Mine" most frequently were more prone to heart attack than those who did not!

One of the most heartening encounters was with the three young American cardiologists who took great interest in the program. These cardiologists could earn about 2000 dollars per hour by performing angioplasty, whereas their hour's commitment to this program could fetch them less than 300 dollars. They were prepared to devote 6 to 8 hours per week to this program. When asked what attracted them to this program, they said that in an hour they might help two patients with angioplasty while in an hour of this program they might help 20 patients and that too probably more significantly.

An Indian cardiologist at Chicago has been investigating the rising incidence of coronary heart disease amongst the young Indians. His research has led him to believe that the growing sense of isolation is a major cause for the increased incidence. Isolation encouraged smoking, drinking, and indulgence in fast foods rich in fat. The prosperity was also responsible for unhealthy lifestyle. During my visit to England at Leceister I had a similar experience. The young Indians below the age of 35 were increasingly falling prey to coronary heart disease.

During my recent visit to the USA, Dr. Robert Pritiken of the Longevity Centre at Los Angeles related to me a case history of a 55 year old patient who had 90% obstruction in his left anterior discending (L.A.D.) coronary artery. The patient was advised angioplasty. However, he joined the reversal of atherosclerosis program at Los Angeles and in a year's time his repeated angiogram showed reduction in the obstruction of the left anterior discending artery by 60%, that is, it had reduced to mere 30%. The patient's clinical condition had improved a great deal. He was practically symptomless. Six months after this recovery, the patient indulged in a heavy meal. He also took a couple of pegs of hard liquor and then after an emotional outburst had a heart attack. This case history clearly demonstrates that even an occasional indulgence in alcohol and heavy fatty meal accompanied with emotional outrage can cause disruption of a plaque and clot formation in an otherwise normal looking coronary artery resulting in a heart attack.

10. FEEDBACKS

In an effort to study the feedbacks of our patients we held a meeting of the spouses of the participants with Coronary Heart Disease who have been attending our program for longer than a year. All these participants had improved a great deal in their clinical status; they were all controlled by the basic long term therapy. Very encouraging three pieces of information emerged from the group discussion with the spouses:

1. All of them observed that there was no special diet for their husbands and their families had adopted a new way of eating and they enjoyed this. There was no sense of deprivation.

2. They did not fear heart disease any more. They were confident that their husbands would continue to do well. In fact, most of them said that they had improved in their general health, and materially also they were not lagging behind.

3. Their husbands became less irrascible. The situations which used to irritate them before, they say, do not upset them now so much. We like to call these 'spiritual gains'; by that we mean that the spirit of the whole family has thus changed for better. These are the qualities of spirit –

fearlessness, acceptance of the new way of eating without missing the old food habits – the new way of living without using tobacco, alcohol, and without getting angry in situations which would otherwise cause irritation. A generous attitude towards colleagues, superiors as well as subordinates; a desire to be helpful; all these attributes blossom forth due to the practice of meditation. I have talked about meditation in detail. One thing it does most to its practitioner is that it teaches the practitioner to live in present moment, to make the most of the present moment. When one is totally engaged in the present moment, time stands still. Most of the stresses originate from the perception of fleeting time, a constant feeling that there is a lot to be done and that the time is short. A very wise Sufi said, "Be busy the whole day, but while retiring to sleep, do not go with the thoughts of what is left to be done next day. No person has ever closed his eyes for ever having done everything what he wished to do." It is human to plan for the future and reminisce the past. There is nothing wrong in remembering the past. But to be occupied with the past and the future in every living moment is to ruin the essence of life which exists always in the present moment only. So it will be good to retire at night with an idea that all things to be done have been done and now as I sleep there is nothing left out.

A male aged 60, who got bypass surgery done in May 1989, felt miserable because within six months of bypass surgery angina recurred and treadmill test became strongly positive. He was advised to repeat angiography. He has been with us since October 2, 1991 and in his own words, "I am a totally different man with a lot of confidence and with the minimum of maintenance medical therapy, and am practically symptom-free." He is one of our most regular participants of the program which is conducted twice a week for an hour in the evenings. Somebody asked him, "Do you not get bored of doing the same ritual for the last four years?" Mr. Mehta replied that in fact he enjoyed it all the more. Every time he did it, it gave him a new sense of relaxation. The whole exercise is like coming home to oneself.

A retired executive of Life Insurance Corporation of India, aged 60, had a heart attack about three years ago, and was advised angiography as his treadmill test was strongly positive. He did not have angiography done. He joined our program in 1993. Now he is fully rehabilitated and has this observation to make about the program: "Doctor, I had a desire to accomplish three things: (i) to be able to give up smoking since I was a chainsmoker; (ii) to be able to reduce weight – I weighed more than 80 kgs., and (iii) to control anger. I was notorious for my bad temper. Now I am happy to say that I have achieved all these. I do not smoke at all. I do not even think of smoking. I have reduced weight by about 10 kgs, and my family is happily surprised at the change of my temperament."

A 35 year old male had a severe heart attack about two years ago (1993). His coronary angiogram showed triple vessel disease. He was advised bypass surgery. Now without surgery he is completely recovered, doing about 12 hours of work in his own small steel furniture factory. He has also changed his food habits. He takes medications regularly and says that he enjoys the visualization techniques and meditation a great deal. He vividly picturises in his mind that the deposits in his coronary arteries have been washed away and the blood flow through his coronary arteries is now completely unobstructed and feels energetic all day long.

Another male about 58 was denied the benefit of bypass surgery because of severe diffuse disease in his coronary arteries. He had angina on even the slightest effort. He joined our program about three years ago. He is now practically symptom-free on modest medications. He walks daily for about 30-40 minutes, rides his two-wheeler, and remains busy with his tailoring business the whole day.

A young coronary patient related his experience in an eye camp where he gave his services as a volunteer for 16 hours at a stretch. During the whole day about 150 cataract operations were done. He had to give even bedpan to the patients. However he did not experience angina on that day whereas during his office work he feels tired even after six hours of routine work and gets angina even if he does moderately strenuous work. This is known as "Helper's High". While helping others the chemical changes that occur in the blood promote health.

The feedback from our lady participants of the age group between 40 and 55 is also very encouraging. A lady aged 52 had severe unstable angina about 3 years ago. She was advised coronary angiography. However, she pursued intensive medical treatment and took the help of our program. Now for the last year and a half she has been practically symptom-free on minimum medication. She keeps busy all day long with her household duties.

Another lady aged 55 had angina about three years ago. She was also advised to go in for angiographic studies. She did not get angiography done. She affirms that she is greatly benefited by the program. She could even bear with equanimity the loss of her dear younger sister due to cancer.

Another unfortunate couple in their late fifties had a great tragedy, for their daughter was murdered. The husband got angina and the wife suffered from angina and severe depression. Both of them have now a sense of well-being, and for their recovery they give credit to the program.

These are sample feedbacks. Since the book is meant largely for the common reader the scientific details of the cases given here are not mentioned. We have now an array of them reiterating the same benefits: freedom from fear, the increased confidence, joy of the new way of life, reduction in anger, the increased feeling of oneness with the people around, and medications reduced to the bare minimum to control their associated hypertension and diabetes, as the case may be. To sum up, we are reasonably convinced that the program has added a new dimension to the healing of Coronary Heart Disease. We would call it a "spiritual dimension", the dimension without which the management of coronary heart disease would be incomplete.

11. TOMORROW'S PRESCRIPTION
FOR CHD

1. Medication
2. Dietary advice
3. Yogic exercises:

a) Abdominal breathing - four times a day, each time for about 10 breaths.

b) Five minutes of *shavasan,* progressive deep relaxation twice a day.

c) Three to five minutes of meditation, three times a day.

4. Advice to attend a centre of yogic exercises, at least twice a week to have the experience in a group.

It is our observation through a detailed study of more than 100 patients who have participated in our program that they feel much less tense and isolated after attending only 6 to 10 sessions. Each session consists of about one hour of light stretching and relaxation exercise of the various parts of the body, leading to *shavasana* and meditation in a group of about 150 participants. A strong point of this program is that it remarkably helps the patients who have severe diffuse disease of the coronary arteries and are considered unfit for surgery. Dr. Dean Ornish mentions that the patients with disabling angina not responding to intensive medical treatment respond quite favourably to the indepth stress management. In fact, he observes that the severer the symptoms the quicker is the favourable response. This may sound a tall claim. However, our experience also more than supports this claim. Moreover, women, on a statistical data who do not do well with angioplasty or CABG, show better results in the heart reversal program than men with CHD. In all situations hence where conventional methods fail, the indepth stress management on the lines of the Universal Healing may prove helpful.

The reader will be happy to learn that our oriental yogic method of healing is now scientifically accepted in about 24 centres in the world. A chain of such heart reversal programs exists in USA, Canada and Australia (List of programs included in the Appendix). These facts deserve wide publicity. Here it may be noted that the indepth stress management in the Universal Healing Program consists of five points and all of them work in unison, each one supporting the other. For example, the practice of meditation helps the participants to adhere to low fat vegetarian diet. The low fat vegetarian diet is congenial to meditation. The light stretching and relaxation exercises leading to efficient *shavasana* in turn, help meditation. Group discussion and sharing of feelings following *shavasana* and meditation are also very effective. Abdominal breathing is by far the simplest and the most effective way to reduce stress. This was borne out vividly by several feedbacks.

The Universal Healing Program during the last four years has collected data from one hundred and thirteen patients out of about two thousand patients who have participated in the program.

A Therapy for Coronary Heart Disease which is effective and that too in a short run and specially more so in those who are not benefited by conventional approach; helpful in making life style changes of smoking cessation and moderation in use of alcohol and acceptance of low fat vegetarian diet; having pleasant side efect like relief from hyperacidity, arthritis, chronic skin disease and insomnia; easily affordable, available everywhere and easy to adopt; having a synergistic effect with any other form of treatment – A therapy with such unique features is the U. H. Program for Coronary Heart Disease.

12. EPILOGUE

We have studied the emotions that damage or poison the heart. We have seen how these emotions change the calibre of the coronary arteries, increase the stickiness of the blood cells (platelets) and viscocity of blood, decrease good cholesterol (HDL) and increase bad cholesterol (LDL) in blood. The total effect may aggravate angina or result in a heart attack. An antidote to these heart toxins lies in the simple yogic disciplines : abdominal breathing, *shavasana* and meditation. We call these disciplines yogic, because they connect the individual to his large Self. They help him to realise his inner strength, his soul force, his real identity.

As adults, we breathe with chest muscles, however, when we practise breathing with abdominal muscles it at once quietens the mind. Breathing is central to all the three yogic disciplines. *Patanjali Yogashastra* intuitively observes that control of breathing controls the restless mind, which in turn controls the circulation. Normally our breathing is involuntary and reflects the state of our mind. If our mind is not at peace, the breathing is rapid and shallow

56

and when the mind is at peace as during deep sleep the breathing is slow, rhythmic and abdominal. So, if we consciously breathe slowly, rhythmically, and abdominally, the mind automatically becomes calm. *Shavasana* is a technique to relax the body which leads to relaxation of the mind. During meditation, one becomes one with the breath, one with the life-force, and this brings about an experience of the soul-force within oneself. The realization of the soul force brings forth the qualities of the soul. They are love, compassion, brotherhood and freedom from the fear of death. It is easy to see that when these qualities develop all the healthful changes occur in the body.

Doctors and their trained personnel can easily teach these techniques in their clinics. Overemphasis or undue strictness in the name of discipline while teaching makes them less effective. An humble attitude of the teacher and a flexible approach bring about good results. The healer ought to heal himself.

APPENDIX A

As part of his efforts to focus establishment attention on the cost implications of not addressing the underlying causes of heart disease, Dean Ornish had met First Lady Hillary Rodham Clinton. He is a member of the office of Alternative Medicine at the National Institutes of Health. The following is an excerpt from a letter Dr. Ornish wrote to Ms. Clinton.

Dear Ms. Clinton,

Please accept sincere and heartfelt appreciation for the opportunity to meet with you on Thursday morning. Thank you for making health care such a high priority in your administration.

In a series of clinical trials conducted during the past sixteen years, funded in part by the National Heart, Lung and Blood Institute of the National Institutes of Health, we have demonstrated that the course of even severe coronary heart disease often can be reversed by a program of comprehensive lifestyle changes without bypass surgery, angioplasty or a lifetime of cholesterol lowering drugs. These lifestyle changes include a very low-fat vegetarian diet, mind-body stress management techniques, moderate exercise, smoking cessation, and psychosocial support.

Comprehensive lifestyle changes may be not only medically effective but also cost-effective in significantly reducing health care expenditures. These choices are most clearly seen in the arena of cardiology, for in no other area are costs so high and the benefits of less costly lifestyle interventions as well-documented.

In the past, lifestyle interventions have been viewed as increasing costs in the short run for a possible savings years later. In this new model, you do not have to wait five years to see a benefit; the reduction in costs is immediate.

Providing lifestyle changes as a direct alternative for patients who otherwise would receive coronary bypass surgery or coronary angioplasty would result in an immediate and substantial cost savings. Last year, over $ 14 billion were spent on coronary bypass surgery in the US at an average cost of at least $ 40,000 per operation, much more when complications occurred. Over $ 5 billion were spent on coronary angioplasty at an average cost of over $ 15,000 per operation. Intensive lifestyle modification is much less costly. For every patient who decides to change his or her lifestyle rather than undergoing bypass surgery, at least $ 40,000 are saved that would have been spent.

Providing lifestyle changes as a direct alternative for patients who otherwise would receive coronary bypass surgery or coronary angioplasty may result in significant long-term cost savings. Despite the tremendous expense of bypass surgery and angioplasty, up to one-half of bypass grafts become blocked after only five years and one third to one-half of angioplastied arteries clog up again after only four to six months regardless of the method used. When this occurs, coronary bypass surgery or coronary angioplasty is often repeated, thereby incurring additional costs.

Rather than the usual course of getting worse and worse over time, many heart patients can get better and better if they make comprehensive lifestyle changes. Within a few weeks, the patients in our research reported a 91 percent average reduction in the frequency of angina (Chest Pain). Most of the patients became essentially pain-free, including those who had been unable to work or engage in daily activities due to severe chest pain. Within a month, we measured increased blood flow to the heart and improvements in the heart's ability to pump. And within a year, even severely blocked coronary arteries began to improve in 82 percent of the patients. They demonstrated even more reversal of heart disease after four years than after one year. Our findings are giving many people new hope and new choices.

Our work is based on the premise that addressing the underlying causes of a problem is ultimately more effective than addressing only its symptoms. Efforts to contain medical costs that do not address the more fundamental causes that determine why people become sick – rather than literally or figuratively bypassing them – will inevitably result in painful choices. This is as true for individual patients as it is with the health care system in general. There is a better alternative.

Our program is now considered a valid alternative, and to a growing number of physicians a clinically preferable alternative to bypass surgery, angioplasty and/ or a lifetime of cholesterol lowering drugs for many patients with moderate to severe coronary heart disease. This approach can provide a third alternative to rationing of continued spiraling costs.

Besides the growing costs, access to bypass surgery is

not equitable. Last year over 90 percent of bypass surgery was performed on white upper middle-class males, despite evidence that heart disease is actually declining in this group whereas it is increasing in women, minorities, and lower socioeconomic groups.

One-half of women are destined to die from heart and blood vessel diseases. Bypass surgery and angioplasty do not work as well in women as in men. Ten times as many women as men die in the hospital; following an angioplasty and women have twice the mortality rate as men following bypass surgery. In contrast, women in our research showed even more reversal of their heart disease than did men. In other words, our program can most benefit those who are most likely to develop heart disease and who have the least access to conventional medical therapies.

My colleagues and I are in the process of training other hospitals in our program, including Beth Israel Hospital in New York and Immanuel Hospital in Omaha. Reimbursement for this program at hospitals that we have trained will enable them to serve those who most need it.

In summary, our research can serve as a model of a "third alternative" in addressing the dilemma of how to significantly lower health care costs and improve access without compromising the quality of health. Clearly, a program that can reverse coronary heart disease would help prevent it for most people. In this context, all Americans may benefit either directly or indirectly.

I admire you greatly and look forward with pleasure to meeting you. With best wishes and warm personal regards.

Sincerely,

Sd/-

Dean Ornish

Q.1 Dr. Kapadia, you've had the highest education in the field of Cardiology in England and America. After such a distinguished career and experience, what really led you to Yoga?

Dr. Medical science has made great progress in the treatment of coronary heart disease. Angioplasty and by-pass surgery are widely used in its management. But neither of them promises a cure. They are palliative measures. Bypass surgery bypasses the problem, as the trouble often recurs.

Over years, I've been looking for an answer. Meanwhile, I came to know of Dr. Dean Ornish's success in the treatment of coronary heart disease through Yoga. In June '91, I got an opportunity to observe his program. It was really amazing to see how in a city like San Fransisco, steeped in materialism and luxury, Dr. Ornish's patients experienced such great relief through Yoga.

Q.2 Could you please tell us about this program at San Fransisco?

Dr. Dr. Dean Ornish's program consists of almost fat-free strict vegetarian diet, modest exercise, progressive deep relaxation *(shavasana),* meditation, group discussions and the sharing of feelings. 40 patients with severe coronary heart disease showed remarkable improvement during 4 years. This was verified by Pocitron Emission Tomography - PET Scan. This is a technique for assessing coronary blood flow to the heart muscle without coronary angiography.

Q.3 Is this Yoga western, or different from what we have here?

Dr. Yoga has its roots in Indian culture. You will be glad to know that Dr. Ornish's program was inspired and evolved by Swami Satchidanandji settled in Virginia who is a disciple of Swami Shivanand.

Q.4 Is it an alternative therapy?

Dr. It is a supportive or supplementary therapy, a nature cure along with medical treatment. It does not replace the traditional therapy.

Q.5 Will you please explain the method of Yoga?

Dr. The purpose of Yoga is to bring about the relaxation of the body and the mind. It is easier to relax the body than the mind. In order to relax the muscles of the body moderate stretching exercises followed by relaxation makes the relaxation process easier. Once the body relaxes, the mind automatically begins to relax. Mind is present in every cell of the body. Hippocrates, the father of medicine, said that there is a measure of conscious thought throughout the body.

Progressive deep relaxation, i.e. *shavāsana* achieved in this manner brings about a relaxed state of mind and body, which prepares the individual for meditation.

Q.6 Doctor, you seem to be turning towards religion.

Dr. Certainly not. Meditation is not a religious ritual. It simply consists in bringing your awareness in the present by focussing on the process of breathing or some sound, like *Om*.

Tension intensifies sympathetic activity which increases heart rate, raises blood pressure, narrows coronary arteries, causes clumping of platelets, often resulting in serious cardiac problems. Meditation retards the sympathetic activity bringing about the dilatation of the narrowed arteries and thinning of blood.

Meditation slows down the rate of "Entropy". In other words, wear and tear are reduced resulting in increase in longevity.

Q.7 How do you meditate?

Dr. The technique is simple. You sit down in a relaxed manner. Close your eyes and simply watch the inhaling and exhaling of your breath. Thoughts may come and go. But remain unconcerned. Breath is life. When you are breathing, it is not only air that you breathe in; you breathe in light and life-force also. Thus your consciousness becomes one with your breath and your life-force, and healing follows.

Out of 16 hours of our waking time, hardly for an hour and a half do we live in the present. Most of the time, our awareness is in the past or the future. Meditation helps us to stay in the present moment. Dr. Dean Ornish says that meditation enabled his patients to change their lifestyle, that is, it made it easy for them to become strict vegetarians and teetotallers.

Q.8 Dr. Kapadia, please tell us something about your replication here of Dr. Dean Ornish's program.

Dr. We started our program on Gandhi Jayanti day, October 2, '91. We meet twice a week on Tuesdays and Fridays in the evening from 6 to 7 p.m. at C. N. Vidyavihar, Ahmedabad. We start with the light stretching and relaxation exercises followed by *shavasana,* meditation and end with group discussion and prayer. A feeling of connectedness fills the air which promotes healing. Isolation breeds disease, connectedness heals. This has been a subject of the recent scientific research in many centres of Europe and USA. The technique evolved in this program to achieve the relaxation of the body and the mind is very simple and effective. The program has a great potential to make the response of the participants to everyday stress healthier. Dr. Dean Ornish has also noted that selfless benevolent work opens up the arteries, whereas self-centredness, hostility, and cynicism are toxic to the heart; they constrict the arteries.

Q.9 It seems, Dr. Kapadia, that you are happy with your program. Have you also scientifically tested the results?

Dr. Our experience is quite encouraging. A gentleman joined us out of sheer curiosity. Within less than six meetings, he gave up his 25 year old addiction to tobacco chewing. A 60 year old male was denied the benefit of bypass surgery as his coronary arteries were so extensively narrowed that the bypass was not feasible. After attending our program for six months he is now leading a normal life.

When 7 of our participants were subjected to EEG test at 11.00 in the morning, our Neuro-Physician was simply astonished to observe their alpha activity. The kind of relaxation it revealed, could not be had normally even after 6 to 7 hours of sound sleep.

This is borne out by another observation that mere three minutes of meditation reduces the oxygen consumption by 20% as against 8% reduction after six hours of sound sleep. A few of our participants have also been able to put off bypass surgery. Those who have undergone surgery, feel happier and more confident after attending our program. Moreover, the program heals the person as a whole.

Our greatest limitation comes from our perception that we are individuals limited in space and time. During meditation, one experiences that one is eternal and boundless. The feeling of connectedness with the universe and wisdom dawns on the individual. This whole experience helps healing in toto. I venture to suggest that if such a program is incorporated in the school curriculum, it could bring about a great change in the human behaviour leading to a saner world.

Q.10 Will you please tell us something more about Yoga and education?

Dr. Oh! This is a very important question. I feel that Yoga in the educational curriculum will complete our education. At the moment, our education is lopsided, largely science oriented. There is nothing wrong with science. We have to know science. But, the true identity of ourselves that is the real knowledge of self is not attained by the pursuit of science. Therefore, in the *Vedas* the knowledge of science is called *avidya*. Let me explain: *avidya* does not mean something against *Vidya*. It is other than *Vidya*. *Vidya* means the knowledge of Self, knowledge of the ultimate reality. Yoga is a synthesis of science and *vidya* or *avidya* and *vidya*. In the *Vedas*, the Rishi says that if you follow *avidya* that is science without *vidya*, you are led into a blind alley. The Rishi does not stop here. He adds, if you follow *vidya* that is knowledge of Self without *avidya* then it is worse. It is complete chaos – *Ghor Andhkar*. In this program the way in which the person learns to relax his body and mind his awareness turns towards the real knowledge - *vidya*. This leads to the healing of the individual as a whole. This is the *summum bonum* of the whole concept of Yoga.

Q.11 Dr. Kapadia, would you please sum up this important topic of heart and Yoga?

Dr. This program is not a panacea or all cure. It does not claim to replace the traditional medical or surgical approach. However, I have no doubt in my mind that it has opened up new, very hopeful frontiers in the management of all stress related diseases like coronary heart disease, high blood pressure, peptic ulcer, arthritis, ulcerative colitis, various skin diseases and many more. This program has a solid scientific basis. It deserves a routine prescription for the treatment of stress related diseases. Moreover, it has a capacity to heal the society as a whole; hence we have named it the Universal Healing Program. Let me end by recalling Dalai Lama's tips to an eminent Harvard Cardiologist, who had gone to Dharamsala to study the benefits of meditation. The quintessence of Tibetan medicine, according to Dalai Lama, consists of three conditions, vital to curing of any disease:

a) The doctor's faith in himself to cure his patient.

b) The patient's faith in his doctor that he will cure him.

c) The doctor's *Karma.*

Thank you Dr. Ramesh Kapadia. Your suggestion that yogic approach could be included in our education program is most interesting. We wish your Universal Healing Program God Speed!

APPENDIX C
Universal Healing A valid third alternative
in the treatment of Coronary Heart Disease

Could a simple technique of relaxation, meditation, modest exercise, vegetarian diet, low in fat, and group support achieve the reversal of coronary heart disease ?

The answer is YES.

Bye bye clogged arteries
Nothing to thrive on anymore !
No meat, no lumps of fat,
No nicotine, no alcohol.
Love dares you, fellowship dares you;
Bye bye clogged arteries,
Nothing to thrive on anymore !

Coronary Heart Disease (CHD) is a global phenomenon. Increasingly more people in the prime of life are victims of this disease in India also. The tell-tale causes of coronary heart disease are : heredity, high blood pressure, diabetes, high serum cholesterol, smoking, and sedentary habits. The way of living and the way of feeling appear to be quite important factors in its rising incidence. Hostility, the lack of social support, and job and family stress are the major causes of heart attack even amongst the young.

The present medical approach is to dilate the coronary arteries and increase the blood flow through them, and diminish the need of oxygenated blood by the heart muscle. The surgical approach is the bypassing of the narrowed arteries or dilating them by inflating a balloon inserted in the narrowed artery. These are palliative measures and do not completely deal with the root cause of the problem.

Dr. Dean Ornish has been conducting a unique program in USA, which has proved a boon to the patients of severe coronary heart disease. He has shown that CHD can be reversed by comprehensive life-style changes. The changes include a very low fat vegetarian diet, the mind-body stress management techniques, moderate exercise, smoking cessation and psychosocial support. Providing life-style changes in this new model as a valid alternative to the patients, who otherwise would receive coronary bypass surgery or coronary angioplasty, results in the immediate and substantial cost savings. In India, bypass surgery and angioplasty cost more than Rs. 1,25,000.00 and Rs. 60,000.00 respectively. Up to one half of bypass grafts may become blocked after about five years, and one third to one half angioplastied arteries may clog up again after only four to six months. When this occurs, coronary bypass surgery or coronary angioplasty is often repeated, thereby incurring additional cost and risk.

With spiralling health care cost, the prevention and less expensive treatment of coronary heart disease ought to be our foremost concern for the teeming millions of our country. We are committed to this goal. The Universal Healing Charitable Trust was founded with an idea of pursuing an all-round approach to the complex problem of coronary heart disease. The main objectives are:

* A holistic approach accommodating all measures – drug as well as non-drug ones of whatever discipline.
* To create mass awareness regarding coronary heart disease, and dispel unnecessary fear of the disease.
* To promote research, and original thinking in the prevention, treatment and rehabilitation of the patients of coronary heart disease.
* To simplify the treatment of coronary heart disease bearing in mind the cost effectiveness of all interventions.
* All the above efforts to be made with the scientific temper without prejudice to the widely accepted current methods of treatment and prevention.

Inspired by the favourable results of Dr. Dean Ornish's program, we launched a program on the similar lines at Ahmedabad on October 2, 1991, the Gandhi Jayanti day.

The program consists of

* Diet counselling
* Moderate exercise like walking on level for 30 to 40 minutes
* Stretching and relaxation exercises leading to progressive deep relaxation, i.e. *shavasana*
* Meditation and Visual Imagery
* Group discussion with emphasis on the sharing of feeling.

Diet

Ordinarily our diet is rich in fats, simple carbohydrates, and contains excess of salt. Fat is almost 30% to 40% of the total calorie intake. It is recommended that dietary fat should not exceed 10% of the total calories. Experts recommend not more than 3 grams of sodium for adults.

Non-vegetarian diet is rich in fat, cholesterol and oxidants which increase the production of free radicals in the body. The excess of free radicals damages body cells, accelerates aging and atherosclerosis, and increases the proneness to heart disease, cancer, lung diseases, and cataract. Hence pure vegetarian diet is recommended. Vegetarian diet being rich in complex carbohydrates has antioxidant properties which reduce free radicals in blood. In our program, a qualified dietician guides the participants regarding proper diet and gives individual advice taking into account the dietetic habits of the family.

Exercise

Regular daily walking on level at a moderate speed for 30 to 40 minutes is all that is recommended.

Shavasana

Shavasana has been practised from the ancient times in different ways. It has been considered the king of asanas. Physical and mental relaxation achieved by *shavasana* has no equal. During *shavasana* slow rhythmic alpha activity is recorded from the frontal lobe of the brain, and various chemical changes occurring in the body promote healing by increasing the immune status of the individual.

Meditation and Visual Imagery (Visualization)

It is difficult to calm the mind even for a few seconds. It is estimated that out of 16 hours of our waking time, hardly for an hour and a half do we live in the present. Most of the time our awareness is in the past or future. Meditation helps us to stay in the present moment. It diminishes the need of oxygen by the heart muscles. Within only three minutes of meditation, 20% of oxygen consumption is reduced as against only 8% reduction in oxygen consumption after six hours of sound sleep.

Meditation brings our awareness into the present by focussing it on the process of breathing as well as some sound like **Om**. It slows down the rate of entropy. In other words, wear and tear are reduced. This results in better health and longevity. The progressive deep relaxation, i.e.

shavasana prepares one for meditation. The technique of meditation is simple. Sit in a comfortable manner and gently close your eyes. Bring your awareness to the process of breathing. Simply watch the inhaling and exhaling of your breath. Thoughts may come and go but you remain unconcerned. Breath is life. When you are breathing, it is not only air that you inhale, you breathe in light and life force also. Thus your consciousness becomes one with your breath and life force, and healing follows. When we try to focus our awareness on the natural process of breathing, various thoughts disturb us and our awareness centres round these thoughts. However, we humans have a unique gift of being able to direct our awareness wherever we wish. Thousand times that the awareness wanders to the thoughts, thousand times it is gently brought back to breathing. This is the essence of meditation. Meditation motivates the individuals to adopt a healthy life-style. During meditation one experiences that one is eternal and boundless. The feeling of connectedness with the universe and wisdom dawns on the individual. This experience helps healing in toto. The perception of real identity and of non-flowing time brings about the desired changes. Our greatest limitation is that we perceive ourselves as individuals limited in space and time. This perception is real but not total. There is another dimension of our reality (our larger self) free from the bounds of space and time, which is the source of our everyday reality (our smaller self). During meditation one experiences the boundless dimension of one's reality. Moreover, no experiment in physics has proved the flow of time (Davis). What we experience as the flowing time accelerates wear and tear. When we experience the eternal present and the real identity, the sense of isolation, self-centredness and hostility comes to an end. Visualization means formation of images in one's mind. It is not wishful thinking or fantasy, both of which are unfocussed and passive, whereas visualization is direct and active. It is a therapeutic use of meditation. During meditation, the patient can visualize the cleaning up of blockages in coronary arteries and resumption of blood supply to heart muscles. It also enables us to forgive one for wrongs done to us and it redeems us of the sense of guilt if any.

Group Discussion and Sharing of Feeling

This is also a useful part of the program. Mere expression and sharing of the problems results in reduction in the stress response and substantially benefits healing.

The occurrence of a heart attack is a dynamic process. All of a sudden, the narrowed arteries become further narrowed due to spasm, and the blood flowing through the artery becomes thick due to the increase in viscosity of blood and clumping of platelets. This is usually the result of extreme sympathetic activity following undue physical and mental exhaustion and stress. A heavy meal, alcohol and smoking aggravate the arterial spasm and the clotting of blood. The practice of *shavasana,* meditation, and change in food habits with avoidance of alcohol and smoking blunt the edge of these harmful reactions and save the patient from heart attack.

Dr. Dean Ornish has noted that self-centredness, hostility, and cynicism are toxins to the heart. They constrict the arteries, whereas selfless benevolent work opens them up. The feeling of isolation is by far the most important factor in increasing the incidence of heart attack in the individuals who are prone to it on other scores. The feeling of isolation and hostility in the cancer-prone individuals triggers the incidence of cancer and also affects the immune system causing psoriasis, arthritis and peptic ulcer.

Results of the Program

In one study by Dr. Dean Ornish, 46 patients of coronary heart disease were randomly divided into two groups of 23 each. All the 46 patients were given the conventional advice and treatment and a diet very low in fat. One group was taught stress management, which consisted of *shavasana,* meditation, and visualization. The results of a twenty-four day studies revealed a significant difference in the clinical improvement between the two groups. The group, which was taught the stress management technique, showed much greater improvement indicated by increase in work performance by 55% due to the improvement in the left ventricular function. There was 20% fall in cholesterol level and 90% reduction in the frequency of anginal attack.

We have a similar experience with as many as about 2000 participants uptil now. In a study of 113 patients, over and above the physical benefits of reduction in the frequency of angina and the increased capacity to work, a very encouraging spiritual gain was observed in the increased confidence and wholesome attitude towards life circumstances. Surprisingly, the fear of death almost vanished in a large number of them.

The program does not claim to be a panacea, nor is it opposed to the conventional medical approach including bypass surgery. It is felt, this program can serve as a model of a **third alternative** without compromising the quality of health.

Expert Opinions

Dr. Larry Dossey, Executive Director, Alternative Medicine, National Institute of Health, USA, writes:

"We have considered heart disease to be purely a physical condition. We have focussed on discovering and eliminating risk factors like elevated cholesterol, high blood pressure, diabetes, cigarette smoking and other minor risk factors. In treating CHD, we have relied almost exclusively on the physically based therapies – surgical procedures, drugs, dietary manipulation, and exercise.

"As valuable as these approaches are, we know that they are incomplete, frequently ineffective, costly, and sometimes hazardous. The other methods such as those employed by the Universal Healing Program, based on the landmark work of Dr. Dean Ornish, have resulted in equal and often superior results with less cost and fewer side effects".

Dr. M. R. Girinath, a senior cardiovascular surgeon of India, writes about the UH Program :

"The incidence of CHD in India has shown steady increase during the last few decades. In contrast, in the western countries there has been a steady decrease in the incidence of this dreaded disease. The opposing trends highlight the fact that we are not paying enough attention to the preventive measures.... Having been active in the management of coronary artery disease, especially with respect to the interventional methods of treatment such as balloon angioplasty and bypass surgery, I am firmly convinced that though these forms of treatment have their own place, prevention is superior to any other form of treatment."

A considerable data on the benefits of low-fat vegetarian diet, *shavasana,* meditation with visual imagery, and group support in reversing Coronary Heart Disease is being collected in a chain of "Heart Diseases Reversal Collaborative Network" at 25 centres in the United States of America, 3 in Australia, 1 in Canada and the Universal Healing Program in India.

Select bibliography

• *Reversing Heart Diseases* • *Eat More, Weigh Less* -
by Dr. Dean Ornish, M.D. • *Space Time Medicine*
• *Recovering The Soul* • *Beyond Illness* • *Meaning &
Medicine* • *Healing Words* - by Dr. Larry Dossey, M.D.
• *Quantum Healing* • *Ageless Body, Timeless Mind* - by
Dr. Deepak Chopra, M.D. • *Primer of Universal Healing*
• *Wealth of Food, Health of Heart* • *Heart Disease : A
New Direction* – by Dr. Ramesh I. Kapadia

UHP Centres

The program is conducted at these centres with the help of audio cassette.

- Rajkot
  (1) Saurashtra High School, Kalavad Road.
  Tuesday to Friday, Evening 6.30 to 7.30
  Contact Tel. No. (0281) 2453122 - 2451215 - 2386017
  (2) Kanta Stree Vikas Gruh
  Monday to Thursday, Evening 6.30 to 7.30

- Mumbai
  (1) Ghatkopar (E)
  V. C. Gurukul Highschool, Tilak Road, Ghatkopar (East)
  Tuesday & Friday Evening 5-45 to 7-00
  Contact : Dhirendra B. Shah
  Tel. No. (O) 25129947 (R) 25137220
  (2) Vileparle(E)
  Nadkarni Kendra Hall
  Play Ground Cross Road No.2, Nehru Road,
  Vile Parle (E)
  Sunday Morning 7-00 to 8-00
  Contact R. N. Shah
  Phone : 28355642
  (3) Matuna (C.R.)
  Kapol Boarding Vidyalaya
  573/574, Khushaldas Parekh Marg, Matunga,
  Daily Morning 7-30
  Contact : Rameshbhai Vyas
  Tel. (O) 24312377 (R) 24098787
  (4) Borivali (W)
  201, Ruchi Apartment, Devidas Lane,
  Behind Raghunath Tower, Borivali (W)
  Daily : Morning 7-00 to 8-00
  Contact : Bipin Parekh
  Tel. (O) 28923447 (R) 28935158, 28930271

77

(5) Santacruz (W)
Charad Smruti Seva Prakalp
2nd Gauthan Lane, Near Bata
Santacruz (W)
Saturday Morning 7-30 to 8-15
Contact : Hinaben Engineer

- Mandal
  Dr. Ramanbhai N. Gajjar, Tel. No. (02715)253257
- Visnagar
  AAPI Preventive Health Clinic
  Dr. J. N. Jhaveri, Tel. No. (02765)231332
- Ahmedabad
  Gajjar Hall, Law Garden
  Sunday & Wednesday 7-00 to 8-00 AM
  Contact : Mehul Bhatt or Ramesh Anadkat
  Tel. Nos. (O) 6565935 & 6430213 Gujarat
  Institute of Civil Engineers & Architects.
- Navsari
  Lion's Orthopaedic Hospital
  Tuesday and Friday, Morning 6-30 to 7-30
  Kumarbhai Shah, Tel. No. (02637)258621

USA
- San Fransisco
  Vasanthi Bhat, Tel No. (408) 257-8418
- Harrisburg
  Girish Modi Tel. No. (717) 732-2426
  Email : girish_modi@hotmail.com
- Los Angeles
  Jay Bhavsar, Tel. No. (909) 949-6266
  Email : kanaidrum@aol.com.
- Dallas
  Surendra Naik, Tel. No. (972) 772-3484
  Email : sbnaik@dallas.net
- Nebraska
  Janak Dave, Tel. No. (402) 292-3790
  Email : janakdave@juno.com
- Jayant Zalavadia, Tel. No. (650) 654-1262
  Email : jayant_zalavadia@yahoo.com

78

OTHER BOOKS BY DR. RAMESH I. KAPADIA

PRIMER OF UNIVERSAL HEALING
The book is an inspiring spin-off of the universal healing program. The technique of *Shavasana* and meditation – as explained in this book – is very simple yet quite effective. It has a solid scientific basis and can be practised by anyone.

Price Rs. 50/-

WEALTH OF FOOD - HEALTH OF HEART
The book opens up a new way for the patients of heart disease to enjoy good health without losing in any way the joy of eating.

Price Rs. 20/-

HEART DISEASE : SCIENCE AND SPIRITUALITY
This book puts forth the role of science and spirituality in the treatment of coronary heart disease.

Price Rs. 25/-

SPINNING ONE'S OWN HEALTH
Spinning One's Own Health deals with the basic tools a person has with him all the time to harness his inner strength to its fullest. We feel confident, the reader will get some insight as to how he can spin his own health by studying this book.

Price Rs. 30/-

HEART TO HEART
This small book clarifies the concepts and benefits of Universal Healing Program.

Price Rs. 15/-

PREVENTION OF HEART ATTACK
The book deals with recent trends in research on prevention of heart attack.

Price Rs.20/-

SHAVASANA : KEY TO HEALTH AND BLISS
This book on Shavasana exemplifies the technique and usefulness of this ancient yogic discipline.

Price Rs.20/-

Publishers:
Navajivan Publishing House, Ahmedabad-380 014 (India)

Dr. Ramesh Kapadia's books available at :

- **Navajivan Trust**, Behind Gujarat Vidyapith,
  P.O. Navajivan, Ahmedabad-14
  Phone : 754 06 35

- **Navajivan Trust**, 130, Shamaldas Gandhi Marg,
  Mumbai-400 002
  Phone : 2201 97 56

- **Sarvodaya Sahitya Mandir**,
  Railway Station, Platform No.1, Ahmedabad-380 001

- **Lokmilap Trust**,
  1565, Sardarnagar, Bhavnagar-364 001
  Phone : 2566402

- **Gujarat Pustakalaya Sahayak Sahkari Mandali**,
  Raopura, Baroda
  Phone : 2422916

- **Gajanan Pustakalaya**, Tower Road, Surat

- **Pravin Pustak Bhandar**, Labh Chambers, Dhebar Road,
  Opp. Muni. Corpon. Rajkot-360 001
  Phone : 2232460

- **Valsad Book Store**, 6/7, Gulmohar Apartment,
  Vasant Talkies, Valsad-396 001

- **Swadeshi Vastu Bhandar**, Ratanbhai, Masjid Road,
  Jamnagar-396 001
  Phone : 2555734

- **Sarvodaya Book Stall,** Railway Platform No. 1,
  Nagpur-440 002

- **Sat Sahitya Shahayogi Sangh,**
  Gandhi Darshan, Exhibition Grounds, Mukaramjahi Road,
  Hyderabad-500 001
  Phone : 4732569

- **Gandhi Book House,** 1-Rajghat Colony,
  New Delhi-110 002
  Phone : 23311714

- **Karnataka Gandhi Smarak Nidhi,** "Gandhi Bhavan",
  Kumara Park East, Bangalore-560 001
  Phone : 2261967

- **Vani Mandir,**
  University Marg, Bapunagar, Jaipur-302 015

- **Khadi Gramodyog Bhavan,**
  844, Anna Salai, Chennai-600 002

- **Sarvodaya Sahitya,** Railway Station, Allahabad-211 001

- **Shanti Ranjan Das,** C/o. Sarvodaya Office,
  C-52, College Street Market, Calcutta-700 007

- **Sarvodaya Book Stall,** Howrah Station, Old Complex,
  Howrah-711 101

- **Dharma Ganga-Gnan Mandir,** C/o. Kantibhai Parikh,
  316, Mahatma Gandhi Road, Pune-411 001
  Phone :656610

The Program is conducted twice a week on Tuesday and Friday from 5.30 to 7.00 p.m. at C. N. Vidyavihar Prarthana Mandir, Ambawadi, Ahmedabad-380 006

•

For further information please contact :

Mr. Nandlal T. Shah
L-43, Swatantrya Senaninagar,
Opp. Nava Wadaj Bus Terminus,
Ahmedabad-380 013
Tel : (079) 7621733

•

Mr. Manikant R. Shah
Tel : (079) 642 2399
Email : greatbapuji@hotmail.com

•

Mr. J. D. Trivedi
Tel : (079) 630 0746

•